The 3 minute, 90 Day Gratitude Journal
for girls

Name ___________________________

Starting Date

Day    Month    Year

___________   ___________   ___________

MY 3 MINUTE GRATITUDE JOURNAL

I am GRATEFUL!

The benefits of the 3 Minute, 90 day Gratitude Journal

Completing a Daily Gratitude Journal helps us recognize the great things we already have in life!

To boost our appreciation for things, it is important to start by writing one or two things down every day that you are grateful for. These can be things that have happened in the past, how far you have come over the past year, current events at school, or something happening in your life right now. To help, it could be things you do with your family and friends like holidays, the achievements you have earned for sport, or anything else you are grateful for.

By taking just 3 minutes each day to reflect on the things in your life that matter to you, it will give you the confidence to make new leaps and bounds for each day. Gratitude is important and something we all need to think of every single day.

I hope you enjoy the **3 Minute, 90 Day Gratitude Journal.**

Wishing you all the best,

Romney Nelson

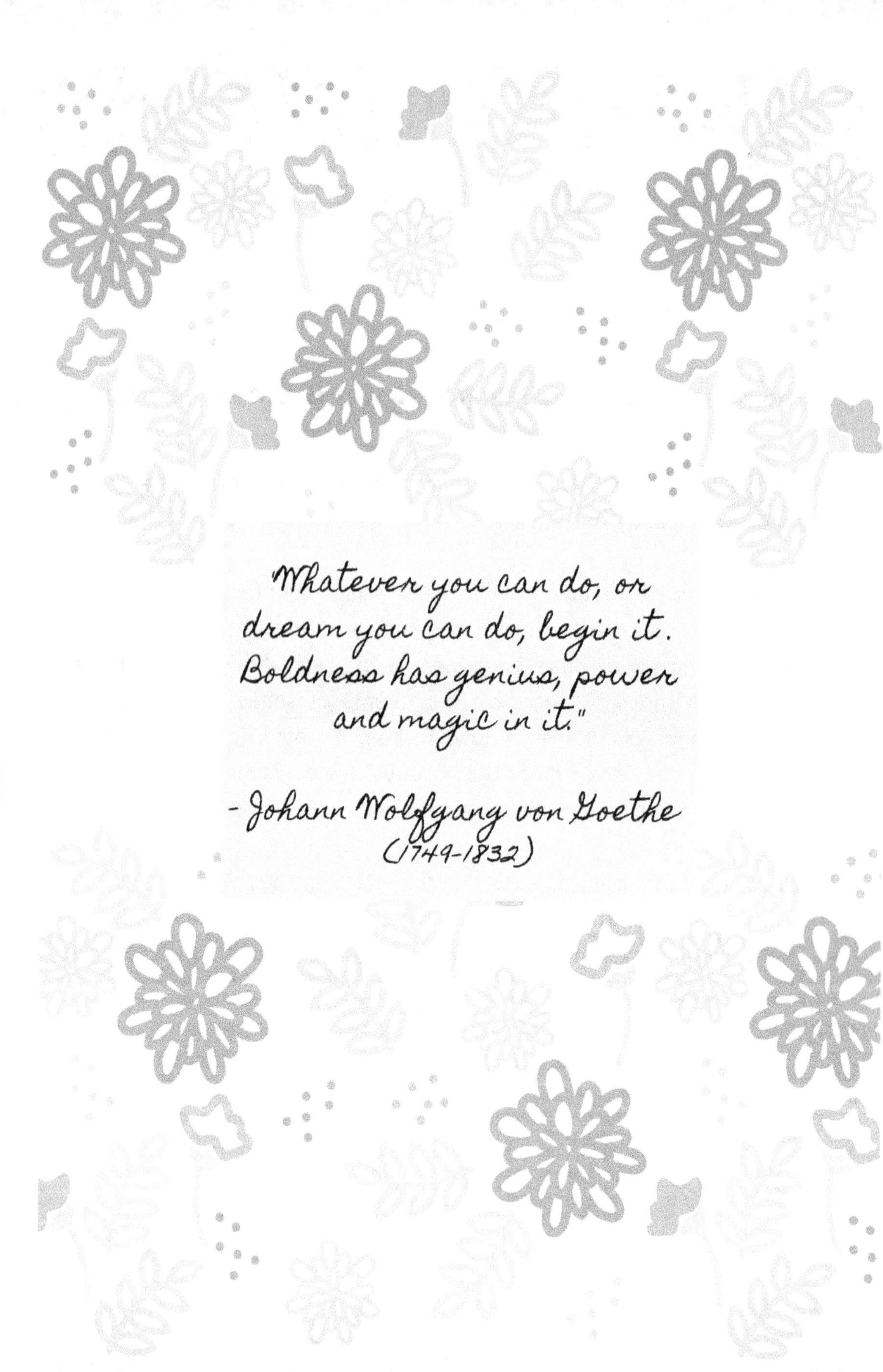
"Whatever you can do, or dream you can do, begin it. Boldness has genius, power and magic in it."

- Johann Wolfgang von Goethe
(1749-1832)

MY 3 MINUTE GRATITUDE JOURNAL

01 **Today I feel**
Tick the face below...

DATE ___ / ___ / ___

TIME ___ : ___

02 **Gratitude.**
I am grateful for...

____

____

____

03 **Complete this sentence**
Today I am looking forward to.......

____

____

____

04 **Today is:**

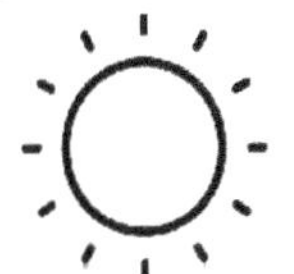

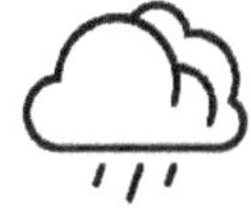
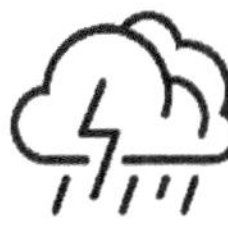

01 **Today I feel**
Tick the face below...

DATE ___ / ___ / ___
TIME ___ : ___

02 **Gratitude.**
I am grateful for...

____

____

____

03 **Complete this sentence**
Today I am looking forward to.......

____

____

____

04 **Today is:**

MY 3 MINUTE GRATITUDE JOURNAL

01 Today I feel
Tick the face below...

DATE ___ / ___ / ___

TIME ______ : ______

 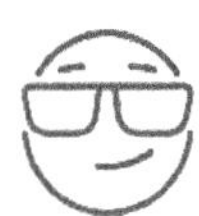    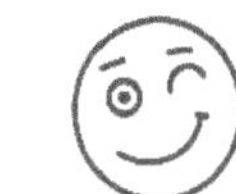

02 Gratitude.
I am grateful for...

____

____

____

03 Complete this sentence
Today I am looking forward to.......

____

____

____

____

04 Today is:

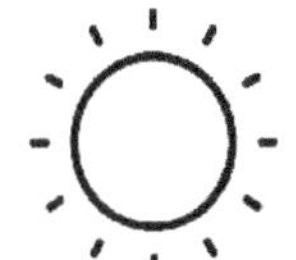  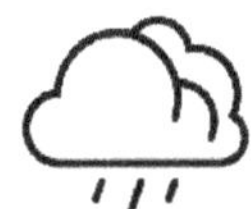 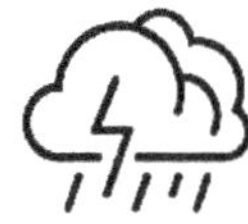  

MY 3 MINUTE GRATITUDE JOURNAL

01 **Today I feel**
Tick the face below...

DATE ___ / ___ / ___

TIME ___ : ___

02 **Gratitude.**
I am grateful for...

____

____

____

03 **Complete this sentence**
Today I am looking forward to.......

____

____

____

04 **Today is:**

MY 3 MINUTE GRATITUDE JOURNAL

01 Today I feel
Tick the face below...

DATE ___ / ___ / ___

TIME _____ : _____

02 Gratitude.
I am grateful for...

____

____

____

03 Complete this sentence
Today I am looking forward to.......

____

____

____

____

04 Today is:

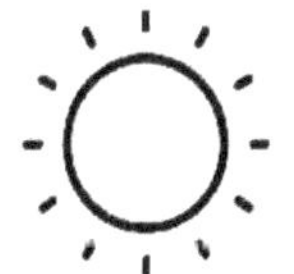

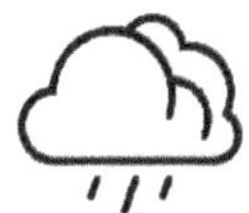
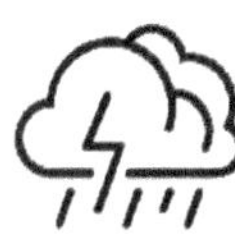

MY 3 MINUTE GRATITUDE JOURNAL

01 Today I feel
Tick the face below...

DATE ___ / ___ / ___

TIME ___ : ___

02 Gratitude.
I am grateful for...

03 Complete this sentence
Today I am looking forward to.......

04 Today is:

01 **Today I feel**
Tick the face below...

DATE ___ / ___ / ___
TIME _______ : _____

 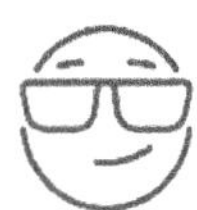    

02 **Gratitude.**
I am grateful for...

____

____

____

03 **Complete this sentence**
Today I am looking forward to.......

____

____

____

____

04 **Today is:**

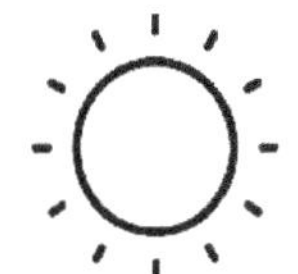  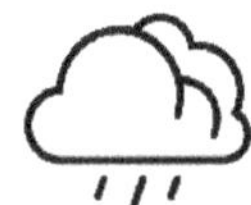 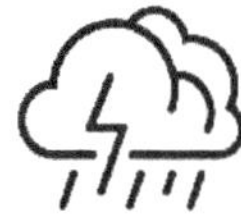  

Congratulations! You have completed your first 7 Days! That's FANTASTIC!

01 Moments

What was your favorite thing you did over the past 7 days?

____

____

____

02 Be Creative!

Draw a picture of something you did over the past 7 days with a family member, a friend or something at school.

MY 3 MINUTE GRATITUDE JOURNAL

01 Today I feel
Tick the face below...

DATE ___ / ___ / ___
TIME _______ : _______

02 Gratitude.
I am grateful for...

____

____

____

03 Complete this sentence
Today I am looking forward to.......

____

____

____

04 Today is:

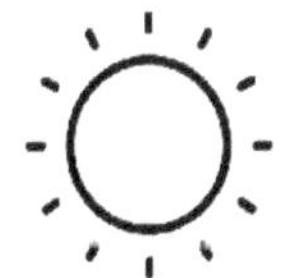  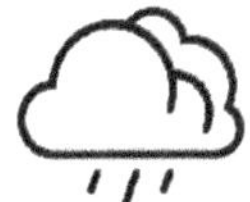 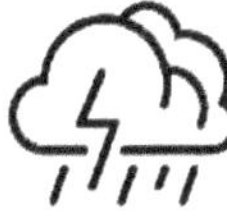  

MY 3 MINUTE GRATITUDE JOURNAL

01 Today I feel
Tick the face below...

DATE ___ / ___ / ___

TIME ___ : ___

02 Gratitude.
I am grateful for...

____

____

____

03 Complete this sentence
Today I am looking forward to.......

____

____

____

04 Today is:

01 **Today I feel**
Tick the face below...

DATE ___/___/___
TIME _______ : ____

 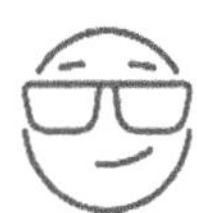    

02 **Gratitude.**
I am grateful for...

____

____

____

03 **Complete this sentence**
Today I am looking forward to.......

____

____

____

____

04 **Today is:**

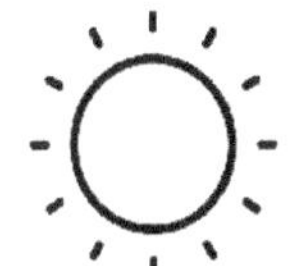  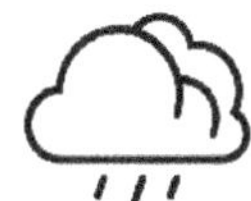 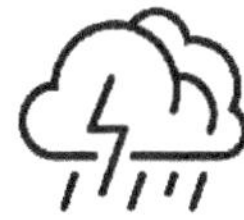  

MY 3 MINUTE GRATITUDE JOURNAL

01 Today I feel
Tick the face below...

DATE ___/___/___

TIME ______:______

02 Gratitude.
I am grateful for...

____

____

____

03 Complete this sentence
Today I am looking forward to.......

____

____

____

____

04 Today is:

MY 3 MINUTE GRATITUDE JOURNAL

01 Today I feel
Tick the face below...

DATE ___/___/___

TIME _______ : _______

02 Gratitude.
I am grateful for...

____

____

____

03 Complete this sentence
Today I am looking forward to.......

____

____

____

____

04 Today is:

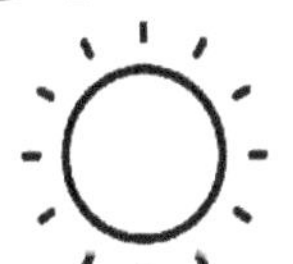

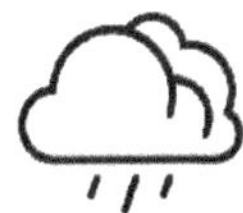
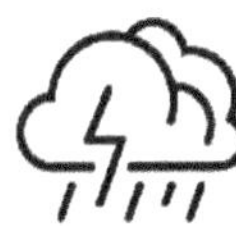

01 Today I feel
Tick the face below...

DATE ___ / ___ / ___

TIME ___ : ___

02 Gratitude.
I am grateful for...

____

____

____

03 Complete this sentence
Today I am looking forward to.......

____

____

____

____

04 Today is:

MY 3 MINUTE GRATITUDE JOURNAL

01 Today I feel
Tick the face below...

DATE ___/___/___

TIME ______ : ______

02 Gratitude.
I am grateful for...

____

____

____

03 Complete this sentence
Today I am looking forward to.......

____

____

____

____

04 Today is:

 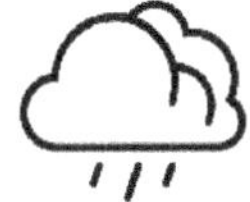 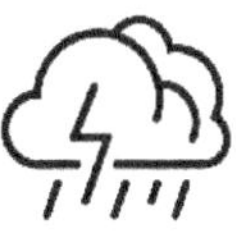  

MY 3 MINUTE GRATITUDE JOURNAL

01 **Today I feel**
Tick the face below...

DATE ___ / ___ / ___

TIME ___ : ___

02 **Gratitude.**
I am grateful for...

____

____

____

03 **Complete this sentence**
Today I am looking forward to.......

____

____

____

04 **Today is:**

MY 3 MINUTE GRATITUDE JOURNAL

01 **Today I feel**
Tick the face below...

DATE ___ / ___ / ___

TIME ___ : ___

02 **Gratitude.**
I am grateful for...

____

____

____

03 **Complete this sentence**
Today I am looking forward to.......

____

____

____

____

04 **Today is:**

  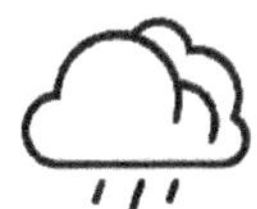 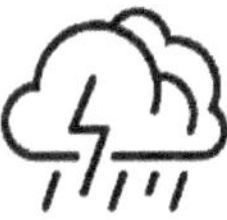  

01 **Today I feel**
Tick the face below...

DATE ___ / ___ / ___

TIME _______ : ___

02 **Gratitude.**
I am grateful for...

____

____

____

03 **Complete this sentence**
Today I am looking forward to.......

____

____

____

04 **Today is:**

MY 3 MINUTE GRATITUDE JOURNAL 

01 Today I feel

Tick the face below...

DATE ___ / ___ / ___

TIME ___ : ___

02 Gratitude.

I am grateful for...

____

____

____

03 Complete this sentence

Today I am looking forward to.......

____

____

____

____

04 Today is:

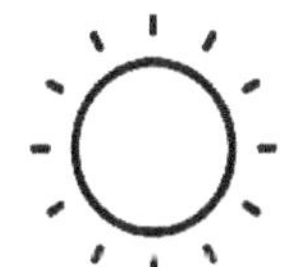  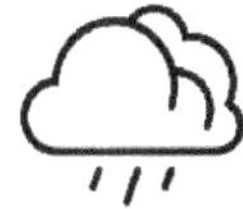 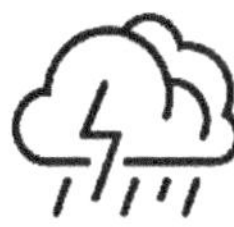  

MY 3 MINUTE GRATITUDE JOURNAL

01 **Today I feel**
Tick the face below...

DATE ___ / ___ / ___

TIME ______ : ______

02 **Gratitude.**
I am grateful for...

03 **Complete this sentence**
Today I am looking forward to.......

04 **Today is:**

MY 3 MINUTE GRATITUDE JOURNAL

01 **Today I feel**
Tick the face below...

DATE _____ / _____ / _____

TIME __________ : __________

02 **Gratitude.**
I am grateful for...

____

____

____

03 **Complete this sentence**
Today I am looking forward to.......

____

____

____

____

04 **Today is:**

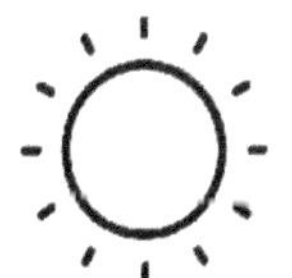  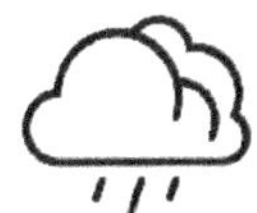 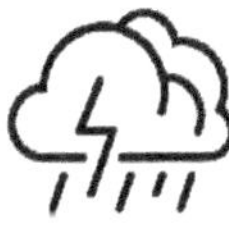  

01 **Today I feel**
Tick the face below...

DATE ___ / ___ / ___
TIME _____ : _____

02 **Gratitude.**
I am grateful for...

____

____

____

03 **Complete this sentence**
Today I am looking forward to.......

____

____

____

04 **Today is:**

MY 3 MINUTE GRATITUDE JOURNAL

01 Today I feel
Tick the face below...

DATE ___/___/___

TIME ______ : ______

02 Gratitude.
I am grateful for...

____

____

____

03 Complete this sentence
Today I am looking forward to........

____

____

____

____

04 Today is:

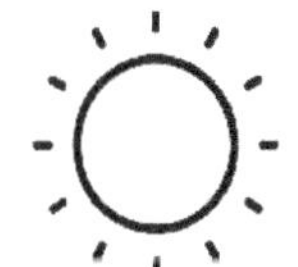

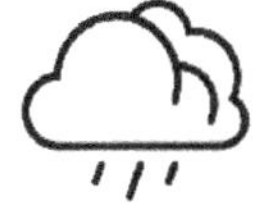
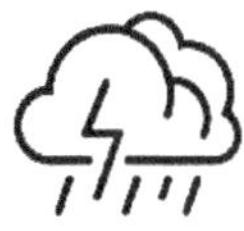

MY 3 MINUTE GRATITUDE JOURNAL

01 **Today I feel**
Tick the face below...

DATE ___ / ___ / ___

TIME ___ : ___

02 **Gratitude.**
I am grateful for...

____

____

____

03 **Complete this sentence**
Today I am looking forward to.......

____

____

____

____

04 **Today is:**

MY 3 MINUTE GRATITUDE JOURNAL

01 Today I feel
Tick the face below...

DATE ___ / ___ / ___

TIME ___ : ___

02 Gratitude.
I am grateful for...

____

____

____

03 Complete this sentence
Today I am looking forward to.......

____

____

____

____

04 Today is:

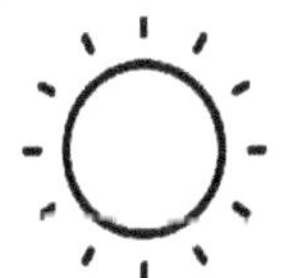

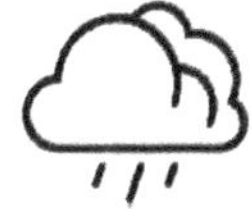
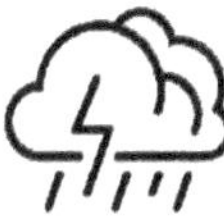
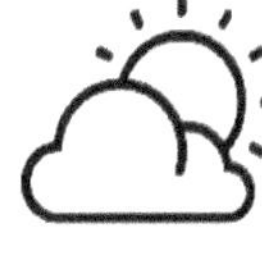

01 **Today I feel**
Tick the face below...

DATE ___ / ___ / ___

TIME _______ : _______

02 **Gratitude.**
I am grateful for...

____

____

____

03 **Complete this sentence**
Today I am looking forward to.......

____

____

____

____

04 **Today is:**

MY 3 MINUTE GRATITUDE JOURNAL

01 Today I feel
Tick the face below...

DATE ___/___/___

TIME ______ : ______

02 Gratitude.
I am grateful for...

____

____

____

03 Complete this sentence
Today I am looking forward to.......

____

____

____

04 Today is:

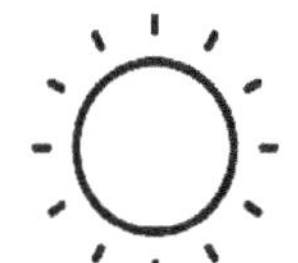

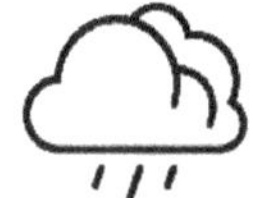
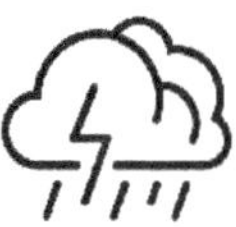

MY 3 MINUTE GRATITUDE JOURNAL

01 Today I feel
Tick the face below...

DATE ___ / ___ / ___

TIME ___ : ___

02 Gratitude.
I am grateful for...

____

____

____

03 Complete this sentence
Today I am looking forward to.......

____

____

____

04 Today is:

MY 3 MINUTE GRATITUDE JOURNAL

01 **Today I feel**
Tick the face below...

DATE ___ / ___ / ___

TIME _______ : _____

02 **Gratitude.**
I am grateful for...

____

____

____

03 **Complete this sentence**
Today I am looking forward to.......

____

____

____

____

04 **Today is:**

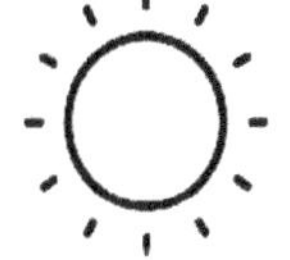
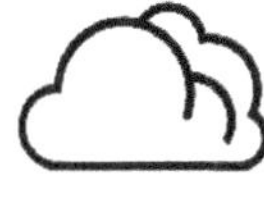
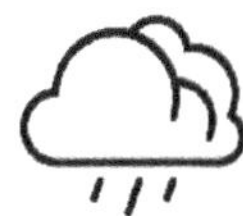
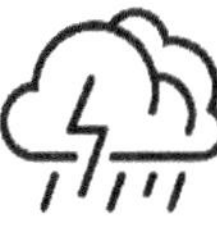
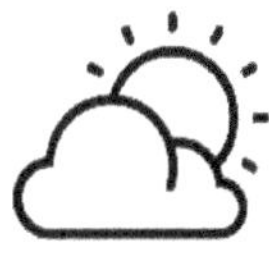

MY 3 MINUTE GRATITUDE JOURNAL

01 **Today I feel**
Tick the face below...

DATE ___ / ___ / ___

TIME ___ : ___

02 **Gratitude.**
I am grateful for...

____

____

____

03 **Complete this sentence**
Today I am looking forward to.......

____

____

____

____

04 **Today is:**

MY 3 MINUTE GRATITUDE JOURNAL

01 Today I feel
Tick the face below...

DATE ___ / ___ / ___

TIME ___ : ___

02 Gratitude.
I am grateful for...

____

____

____

03 Complete this sentence
Today I am looking forward to.......

____

____

____

____

04 Today is:

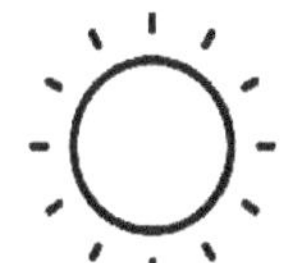

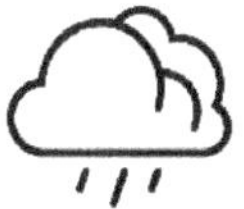
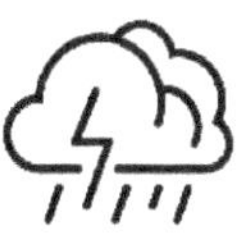

Congratulations! You are up to day 30.

It's time for you to look back over your gratitude journal and answer the following questions.

01 Moments

What were your favorite 3 things you did over the past 30 days?

1.

2.

3.

02 Be Creative!

Draw a picture or stick a photo here that was a special moment for you over the past 30 days.

"We don't remember days; we
remember moments."
- Cesare Pavese
(1908-1950)

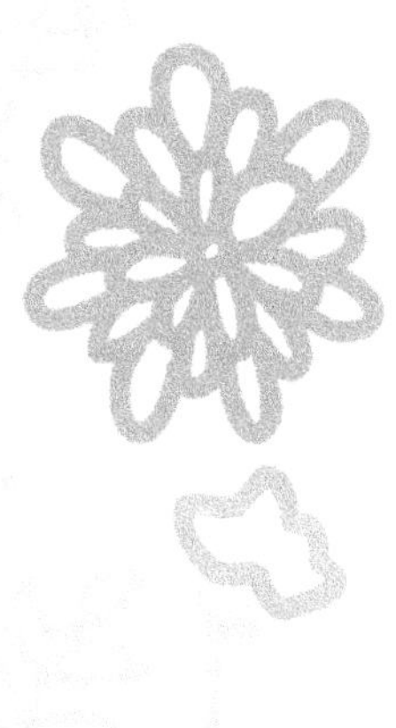
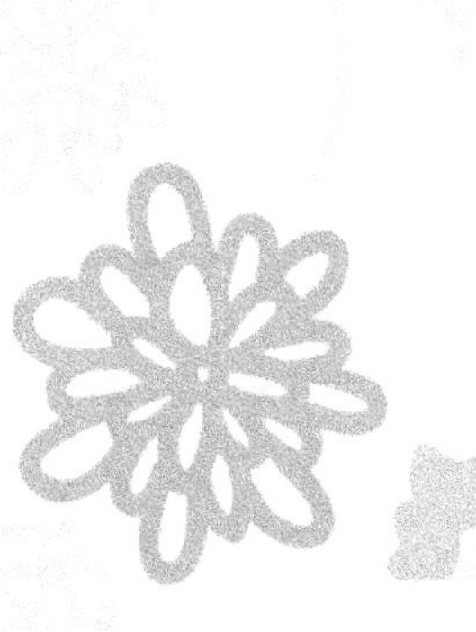
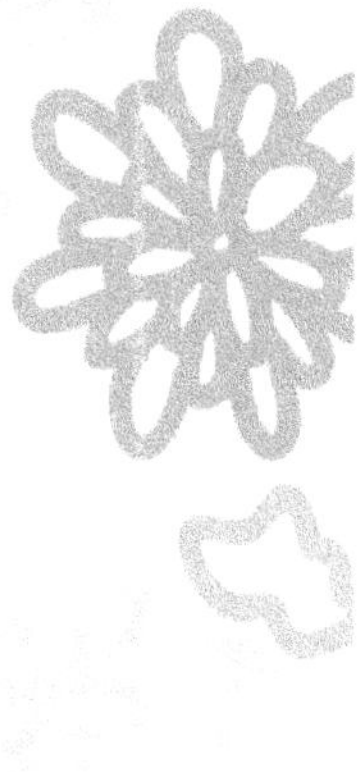

MY 3 MINUTE GRATITUDE JOURNAL

01 **Today I feel**
Tick the face below...

DATE ___ / ___ / ___
TIME ___ : ___

02 **Gratitude.**
I am grateful for...

____

____

____

03 **Complete this sentence**
Today I am looking forward to.......

____

____

____

____

04 **Today is:**

MY 3 MINUTE GRATITUDE JOURNAL

01 Today I feel
Tick the face below...

DATE ___/___/___

TIME ______ : ______

02 Gratitude.
I am grateful for...

____

____

____

03 Complete this sentence
Today I am looking forward to.......

____

____

____

____

04 Today is:

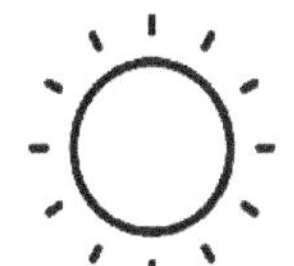

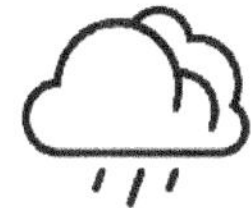
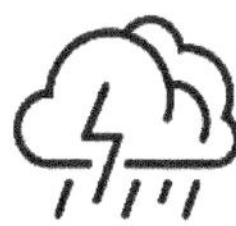

01 Today I feel
Tick the face below...

DATE ___ / ___ / ___

TIME _______ : _____

02 Gratitude.
I am grateful for...

____

____

____

03 Complete this sentence
Today I am looking forward to.......

____

____

____

____

04 Today is:

MY 3 MINUTE GRATITUDE JOURNAL

01 Today I feel
Tick the face below...

DATE ___/___/___

TIME ______:______

02 Gratitude.
I am grateful for...

____

____

____

03 Complete this sentence
Today I am looking forward to........

____

____

____

04 Today is:

MY 3 MINUTE GRATITUDE JOURNAL

01 Today I feel

Tick the face below...

DATE ___ / ___ / ___

TIME _______ : _____

02 Gratitude.

I am grateful for...

____

____

____

03 Complete this sentence

Today I am looking forward to.......

____

____

____

____

04 Today is:

MY 3 MINUTE GRATITUDE JOURNAL

01 Today I feel
Tick the face below...

DATE ___ / ___ / ___

TIME ___ : ___

02 Gratitude.
I am grateful for...

____

____

____

03 Complete this sentence
Today I am looking forward to.......

____

____

____

04 Today is:

MY 3 MINUTE GRATITUDE JOURNAL

01 **Today I feel**
Tick the face below...

DATE ___ / ___ / ___

TIME ______ : ______

02 **Gratitude.**
I am grateful for...

____

____

____

03 **Complete this sentence**
Today I am looking forward to.......

____

____

____

____

04 **Today is:**

MY 3 MINUTE GRATITUDE JOURNAL

01 Today I feel
Tick the face below...

DATE ___ / ___ / ___

TIME ______ : ______

02 Gratitude.
I am grateful for...

____

____

____

03 Complete this sentence
Today I am looking forward to.......

____

____

____

____

04 Today is:

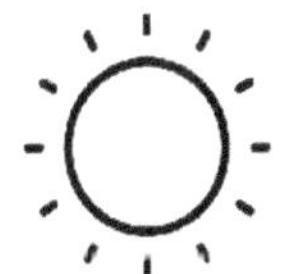

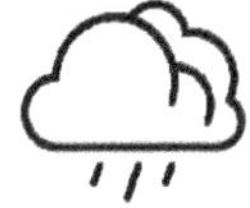
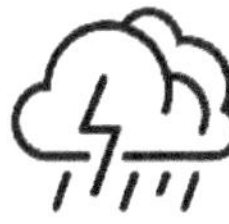

01 **Today I feel**
Tick the face below…

DATE ___ / ___ / ___

TIME ______ : ______

02 **Gratitude.**
I am grateful for…

____

____

____

03 **Complete this sentence**
Today I am looking forward to.......

____

____

____

____

04 **Today is:**

01 Today I feel
Tick the face below...

DATE ___ / ___ / ___

TIME ___ : ___

02 Gratitude.
I am grateful for...

____

____

____

03 Complete this sentence
Today I am looking forward to.......

____

____

____

____

04 Today is:

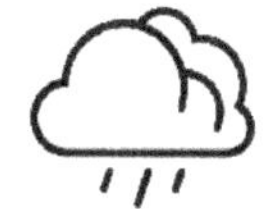
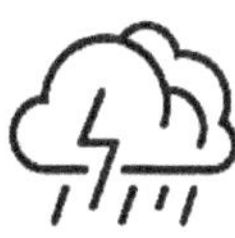
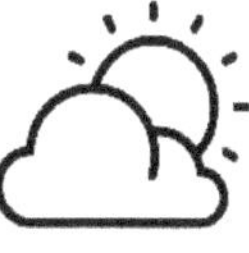

MY 3 MINUTE GRATITUDE JOURNAL

01 Today I feel
Tick the face below...

DATE ___ / ___ / ___

TIME ______ : ______

02 Gratitude.
I am grateful for...

____

____

____

03 Complete this sentence
Today I am looking forward to.......

____

____

____

____

04 Today is:

MY 3 MINUTE GRATITUDE JOURNAL

01 Today I feel
Tick the face below...

DATE ___ / ___ / ___

TIME _______ : _______

02 Gratitude.
I am grateful for...

____

____

____

03 Complete this sentence
Today I am looking forward to.......

____

____

____

04 Today is:

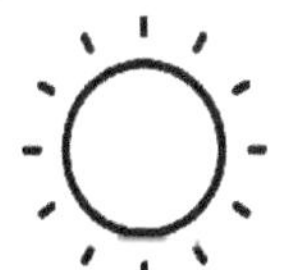

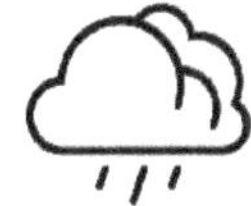
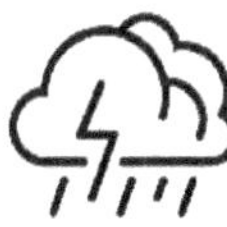

01 **Today I feel**
Tick the face below...

DATE ___ / ___ / ___
TIME ___ : ___

02 **Gratitude.**
I am grateful for...

____

____

____

03 **Complete this sentence**
Today I am looking forward to.......

____

____

____

04 **Today is:**

MY 3 MINUTE GRATITUDE JOURNAL

01 **Today I feel**
Tick the face below...

DATE ___ / ___ / ___

TIME ___ : ___

02 **Gratitude.**
I am grateful for...

____

____

____

03 **Complete this sentence**
Today I am looking forward to.......

____

____

____

____

04 **Today is:**

MY 3 MINUTE GRATITUDE JOURNAL

01 Today I feel
Tick the face below...

DATE ___ / ___ / ___

TIME ___ : ___

02 Gratitude.
I am grateful for...

____

____

____

03 Complete this sentence
Today I am looking forward to.......

____

____

____

____

04 Today is:

MY 3 MINUTE GRATITUDE JOURNAL

01 Today I feel
Tick the face below...

DATE ___ / ___ / ___

TIME ___ : ___

02 Gratitude.
I am grateful for...

____

____

____

03 Complete this sentence
Today I am looking forward to.......

____

____

____

____

04 Today is:

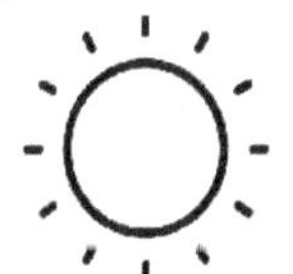  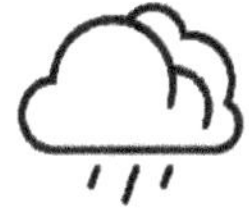 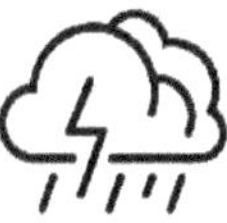  

MY 3 MINUTE GRATITUDE JOURNAL

01 Today I feel
Tick the face below...

DATE ___ / ___ / ___

TIME ______ : ______

02 Gratitude.
I am grateful for...

____

____

____

03 Complete this sentence
Today I am looking forward to.......

____

____

____

____

04 Today is:

MY 3 MINUTE GRATITUDE JOURNAL

01 Today I feel
Tick the face below...

DATE ___ / ___ / ___

TIME ___ : ___

 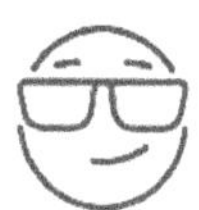    

02 Gratitude.
I am grateful for...

____

____

____

03 Complete this sentence
Today I am looking forward to.......

____

____

____

04 Today is:

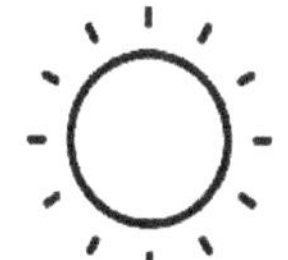  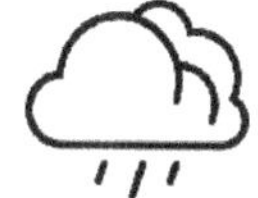 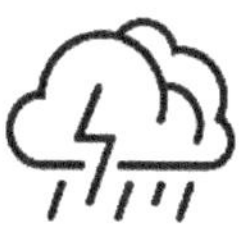  

MY 3 MINUTE GRATITUDE JOURNAL

01 Today I feel
Tick the face below...

DATE ___/___/___

TIME ______:______

02 Gratitude.
I am grateful for...

____

____

____

03 Complete this sentence
Today I am looking forward to.......

____

____

____

____

04 Today is:

MY 3 MINUTE GRATITUDE JOURNAL

01 Today I feel
Tick the face below...

DATE ___ / ___ / ___

TIME _______ : _______

02 Gratitude.
I am grateful for...

____

____

____

03 Complete this sentence
Today I am looking forward to.......

____

____

____

04 Today is:

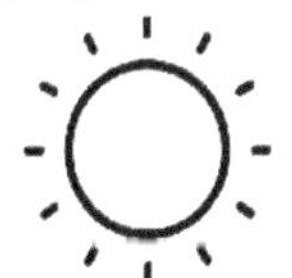 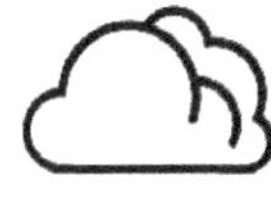 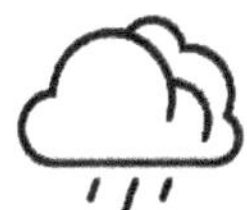 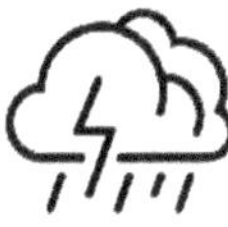  

MY 3 MINUTE GRATITUDE JOURNAL

01 **Today I feel**
Tick the face below...

DATE ___/___/___

TIME ______:______

02 **Gratitude.**
I am grateful for...

____

____

____

03 **Complete this sentence**
Today I am looking forward to.......

____

____

____

____

04 **Today is:**

MY 3 MINUTE GRATITUDE JOURNAL

01 **Today I feel**
Tick the face below...

DATE ___ / ___ / ___

TIME _______ : _______

02 **Gratitude.**
I am grateful for...

____

____

____

03 **Complete this sentence**
Today I am looking forward to.......

____

____

____

____

04 **Today is:**

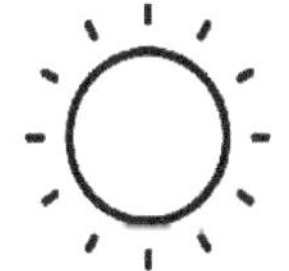  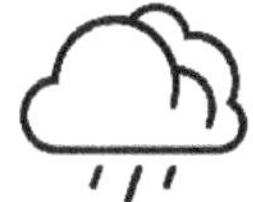 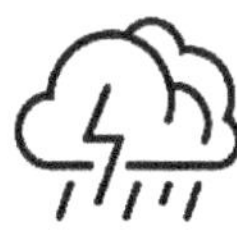  

MY 3 MINUTE GRATITUDE JOURNAL

01 Today I feel
Tick the face below...

DATE ___ / ___ / ___

TIME ___ : ___

02 Gratitude.
I am grateful for...

____

____

____

03 Complete this sentence
Today I am looking forward to.......

____

____

____

____

04 Today is:

MY 3 MINUTE GRATITUDE JOURNAL

01 **Today I feel**
Tick the face below...

DATE ___ / ___ / ___
TIME _______ : _______

02 **Gratitude.**
I am grateful for...

____

____

____

03 **Complete this sentence**
Today I am looking forward to.......

____

____

____

04 **Today is:**

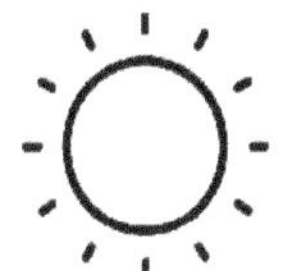  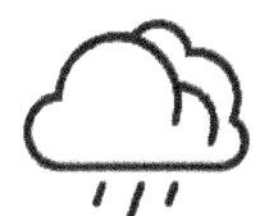 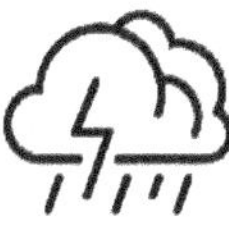  

MY 3 MINUTE GRATITUDE JOURNAL

01 **Today I feel**
Tick the face below...

DATE ___ / ___ / ___

TIME ___ : ___

02 **Gratitude.**
I am grateful for...

____

____

____

03 **Complete this sentence**
Today I am looking forward to........

____

____

____

04 **Today is:**

MY 3 MINUTE GRATITUDE JOURNAL

01 **Today I feel**
Tick the face below...

DATE ___ / ___ / ___

TIME ___ : ___

02 **Gratitude.**
I am grateful for...

____

____

____

03 **Complete this sentence**
Today I am looking forward to.......

____

____

____

04 **Today is:**

01 Today I feel
Tick the face below...

DATE ___/___/___

TIME ______ : ______

02 Gratitude.
I am grateful for...

____

____

____

03 Complete this sentence
Today I am looking forward to.......

____

____

____

04 Today is:

MY 3 MINUTE GRATITUDE JOURNAL

01

Today I feel
Tick the face below...

DATE ___/___/___

TIME ______ : ______

02

Gratitude.
I am grateful for...

____

____

____

03

Complete this sentence
Today I am looking forward to.......

____

____

____

____

04

Today is:

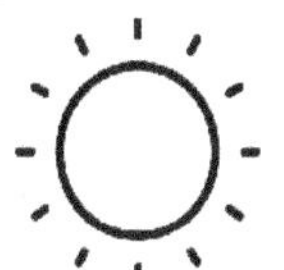  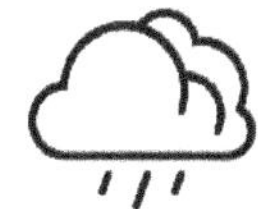 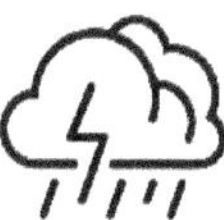  

MY 3 MINUTE GRATITUDE JOURNAL

01 **Today I feel**
Tick the face below...

DATE ___ / ___ / ___

TIME ___ : ___

02 **Gratitude.**
I am grateful for...

____

____

____

03 **Complete this sentence**
Today I am looking forward to.......

____

____

____

____

04 **Today is:**

MY 3 MINUTE GRATITUDE JOURNAL

01 Today I feel
Tick the face below...

DATE ___/___/___

TIME _______:_______

 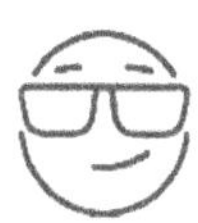    

02 Gratitude.
I am grateful for...

____

____

____

03 Complete this sentence
Today I am looking forward to.......

____

____

____

____

04 Today is:

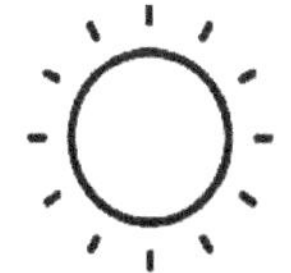  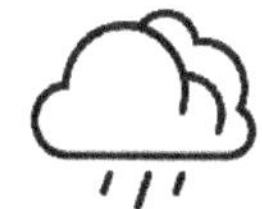 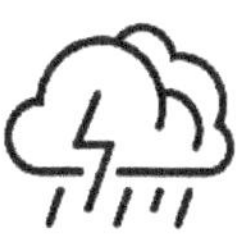  

MY 3 MINUTE GRATITUDE JOURNAL

Congratulations! You are up to day 60.

It's time for you to look back over your gratitude journal and answer the following questions.

01 Moments

What were your favorite 3 things you did over the past 30 days?

1.

2.

3.

02 Be Creative!

Draw a picture or stick a photo here that was a special moment for you over the past 30 days.

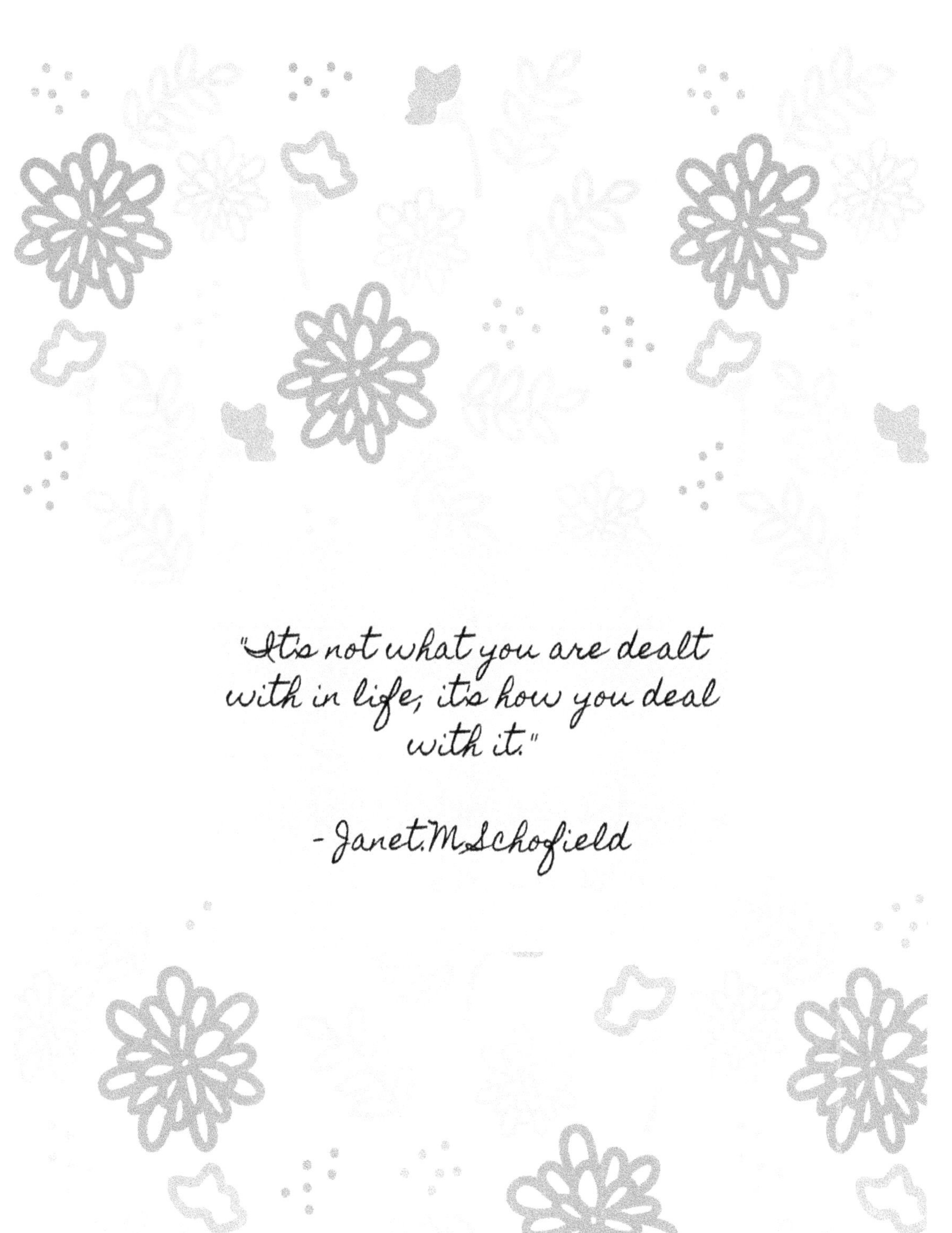

"It's not what you are dealt
with in life; it's how you deal
with it."

- Janet.M.Schofield

01 Today I feel
Tick the face below...

DATE ___/___/___
TIME ___ : ___

02 Gratitude.
I am grateful for...

____

____

____

03 Complete this sentence
Today I am looking forward to.......

____

____

____

04 Today is:

MY 3 MINUTE GRATITUDE JOURNAL

01 **Today I feel**
Tick the face below...

DATE ___ / ___ / ___

TIME ______ : ______

02 **Gratitude.**
I am grateful for...

____

____

____

03 **Complete this sentence**
Today I am looking forward to.......

____

____

____

04 **Today is:**

MY 3 MINUTE GRATITUDE JOURNAL

01 Today I feel
Tick the face below...

DATE ___/___/___

TIME ______ : ______

02 Gratitude.
I am grateful for...

____

____

____

03 Complete this sentence
Today I am looking forward to........

____

____

____

____

04 Today is:

MY 3 MINUTE GRATITUDE JOURNAL

01 Today I feel
Tick the face below...

DATE ___ / ___ / ___

TIME _______ : _______

02 Gratitude.
I am grateful for...

____

____

____

03 Complete this sentence
Today I am looking forward to.......

____

____

____

04 Today is:

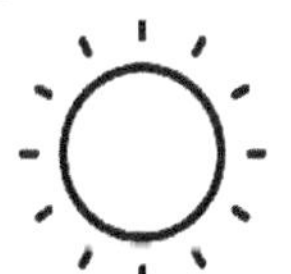

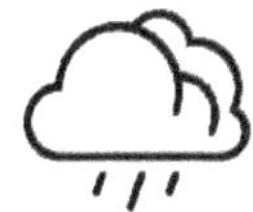
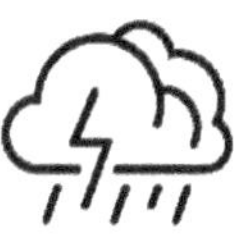

MY 3 MINUTE GRATITUDE JOURNAL

01 **Today I feel**
Tick the face below...

DATE ___ / ___ / ___

TIME ___ : ___

02 **Gratitude.**
I am grateful for...

____

____

____

03 **Complete this sentence**
Today I am looking forward to.......

____

____

____

04 **Today is:**

01 Today I feel
Tick the face below...

DATE ___/___/___

TIME ______ : ______

02 Gratitude.
I am grateful for...

____

____

____

03 Complete this sentence
Today I am looking forward to.......

____

____

____

04 Today is:

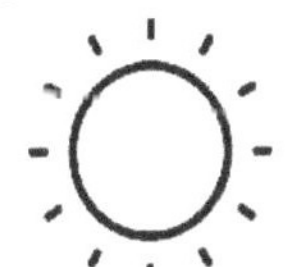  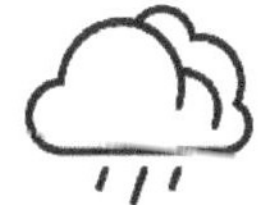 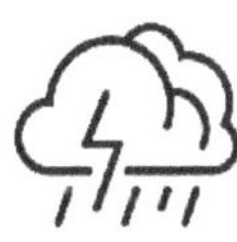  

01 Today I feel
Tick the face below...

DATE ___ / ___ / ___

TIME _______ : _______

02 Gratitude.
I am grateful for...

____

____

____

03 Complete this sentence
Today I am looking forward to.......

____

____

____

04 Today is:

MY 3 MINUTE GRATITUDE JOURNAL

01 **Today I feel**
Tick the face below...

DATE ___/___/___

TIME _______ : _____

02 **Gratitude.**
I am grateful for...

____

____

____

03 **Complete this sentence**
Today I am looking forward to.......

____

____

____

04 **Today is:**

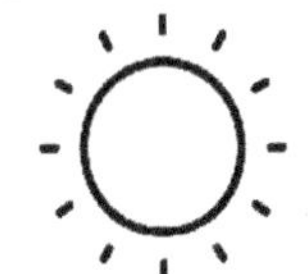  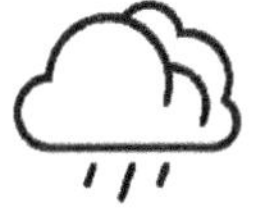 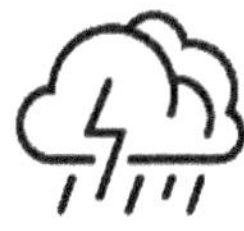  

MY 3 MINUTE GRATITUDE JOURNAL

01 **Today I feel**
Tick the face below...

DATE ___/___/___

TIME ___:___

02 **Gratitude.**
I am grateful for...

03 **Complete this sentence**
Today I am looking forward to.......

04 **Today is:**

MY 3 MINUTE GRATITUDE JOURNAL 

01 Today I feel
Tick the face below...

DATE ___ / ___ / ___

TIME ___ : ___

02 Gratitude.
I am grateful for...

____

____

____

03 Complete this sentence
Today I am looking forward to.......

____

____

____

04 Today is:

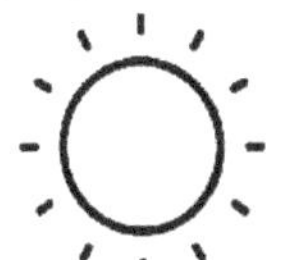  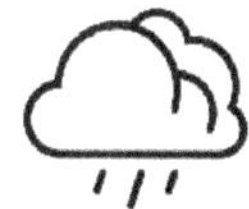 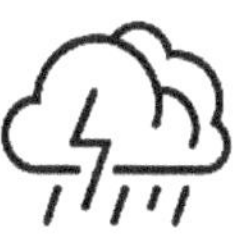  

MY 3 MINUTE GRATITUDE JOURNAL

01 Today I feel
Tick the face below...

DATE ___ / ___ / ___

TIME _______ : _______

02 Gratitude.
I am grateful for...

____

____

____

03 Complete this sentence
Today I am looking forward to.......

____

____

____

____

04 Today is:

01 Today I feel
Tick the face below...

DATE ___/___/___

TIME _______ : _______

02 Gratitude.
I am grateful for...

____

____

____

03 Complete this sentence
Today I am looking forward to.......

____

____

____

____

04 Today is:

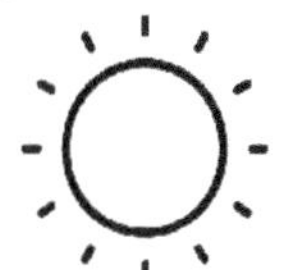

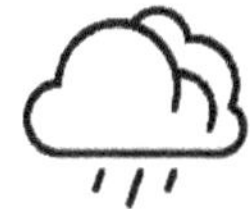
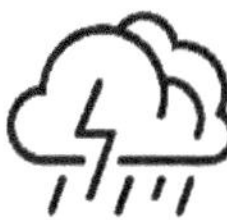

01 Today I feel
Tick the face below...

DATE ___ / ___ / ___

TIME ___ : ___

02 Gratitude.
I am grateful for...

____

____

____

03 Complete this sentence
Today I am looking forward to.......

____

____

____

____

04 Today is:

MY 3 MINUTE GRATITUDE JOURNAL

01 **Today I feel**
Tick the face below...

DATE _____/_____/_____

TIME __________:__________

 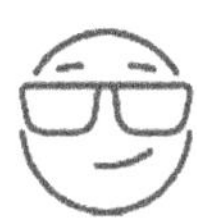    

02 **Gratitude.**
I am grateful for...

____

____

____

03 **Complete this sentence**
Today I am looking forward to.......

____

____

____

04 **Today is:**

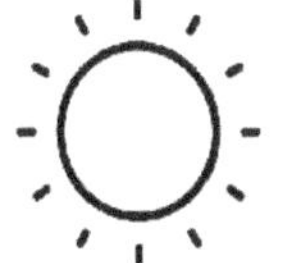  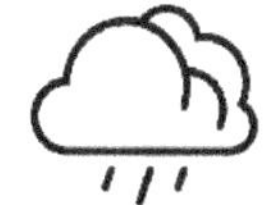 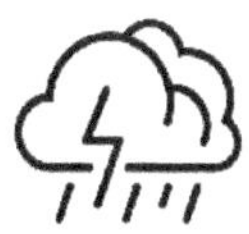  

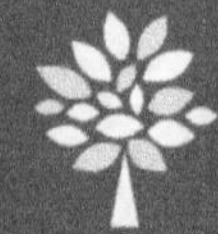

01 **Today I feel**
Tick the face below...

DATE ___ / ___ / ___
TIME _______ : _______

02 **Gratitude.**
I am grateful for...

____

____

____

03 **Complete this sentence**
Today I am looking forward to.......

____

____

____

04 **Today is:**

MY 3 MINUTE GRATITUDE JOURNAL

01 Today I feel
Tick the face below...

DATE ___/___/___

TIME _______ : _______

02 Gratitude.
I am grateful for...

____

____

____

03 Complete this sentence
Today I am looking forward to.......

____

____

____

____

04 Today is:

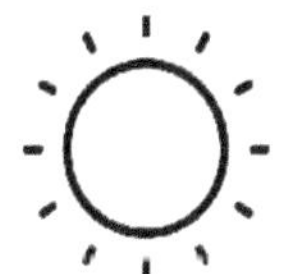  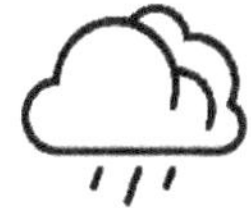 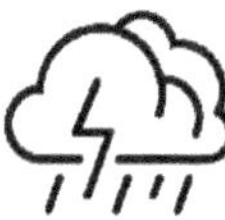  

01 **Today I feel**
Tick the face below...

DATE ___ / ___ / ___
TIME _____ : _____

02 **Gratitude.**
I am grateful for...

____

____

____

03 **Complete this sentence**
Today I am looking forward to.......

____

____

____

04 **Today is:**

MY 3 MINUTE GRATITUDE JOURNAL

01 Today I feel
Tick the face below...

DATE ___ / ___ / ___

TIME _______ : _____

02 Gratitude.
I am grateful for...

____

____

____

03 Complete this sentence
Today I am looking forward to.......

____

____

____

04 Today is:

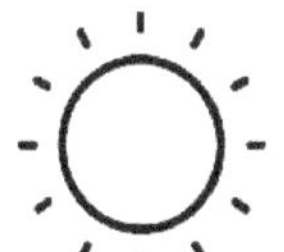  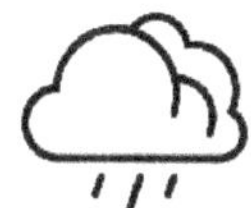 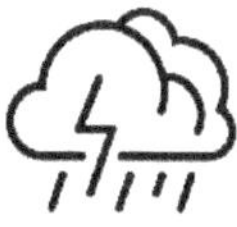 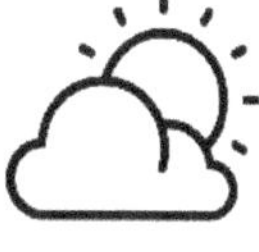 

01 Today I feel
Tick the face below...

DATE ___ / ___ / ___

TIME ___ : ___

02 Gratitude.
I am grateful for...

____

____

____

03 Complete this sentence
Today I am looking forward to.......

____

____

____

04 Today is:

01 Today I feel
Tick the face below...

DATE ___/___/___

TIME _______ : _______

02 Gratitude.
I am grateful for...

____

____

____

03 Complete this sentence
Today I am looking forward to.......

____

____

____

____

04 Today is:

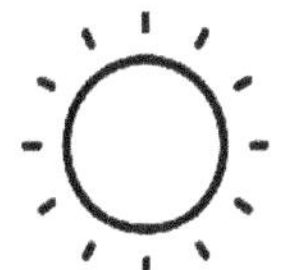  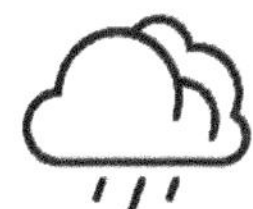 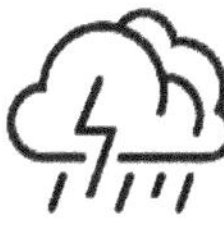  

MY 3 MINUTE GRATITUDE JOURNAL

01 **Today I feel**
Tick the face below...

DATE _____ / _____ / _____

TIME _____ : _____

02 **Gratitude.**
I am grateful for...

____

____

____

03 **Complete this sentence**
Today I am looking forward to.......

____

____

____

04 **Today is:**

MY 3 MINUTE GRATITUDE JOURNAL

01 **Today I feel**
Tick the face below...

DATE ___ / ___ / ___
TIME _______ : _______

02 **Gratitude.**
I am grateful for...

____

____

____

03 **Complete this sentence**
Today I am looking forward to.......

____

____

____

04 **Today is:**

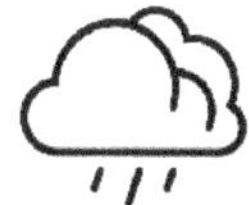
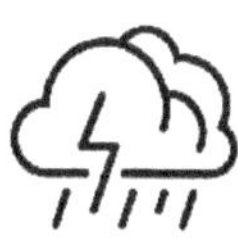
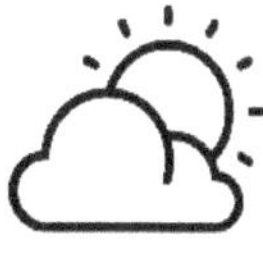

01 Today I feel
Tick the face below...

DATE ___ / ___ / ___

TIME _______ : ______

02 Gratitude.
I am grateful for...

____

____

____

03 Complete this sentence
Today I am looking forward to.......

____

____

____

04 Today is:

01 **Today I feel**
Tick the face below...

DATE ___/___/___

TIME _______ : _______

02 **Gratitude.**
I am grateful for...

____

____

____

03 **Complete this sentence**
Today I am looking forward to.......

____

____

____

04 **Today is:**

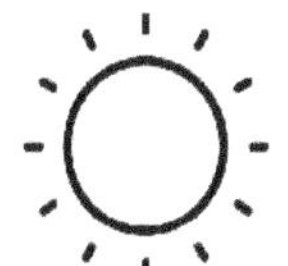  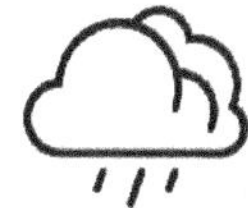 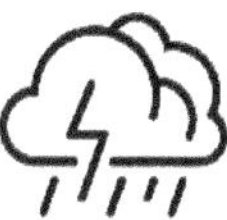  

MY 3 MINUTE GRATITUDE JOURNAL

01 **Today I feel**
Tick the face below...

DATE ___ / ___ / ___

TIME ___ : ___

02 **Gratitude.**
I am grateful for...

____

____

____

03 **Complete this sentence**
Today I am looking forward to.......

____

____

____

____

04 **Today is:**

MY 3 MINUTE GRATITUDE JOURNAL

01 Today I feel
Tick the face below...

DATE ___/___/___

TIME ______ : ______

02 Gratitude.
I am grateful for...

____

____

____

03 Complete this sentence
Today I am looking forward to.......

____

____

____

____

04 Today is:

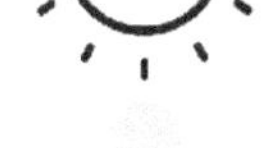

01 **Today I feel**
Tick the face below...

DATE ___ / ___ / ___

TIME _______ : _______

02 **Gratitude.**
I am grateful for...

____

____

____

03 **Complete this sentence**
Today I am looking forward to.......

____

____

____

____

04 **Today is:**

MY 3 MINUTE GRATITUDE JOURNAL

01 Today I feel
Tick the face below...

DATE ___/___/___

TIME ______ : ______

02 Gratitude.
I am grateful for...

____

____

____

03 Complete this sentence
Today I am looking forward to.......

____

____

____

04 Today is:

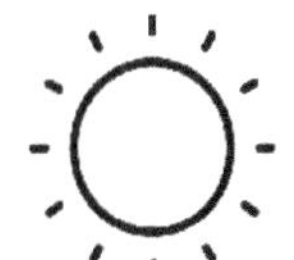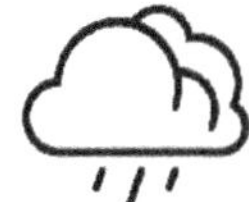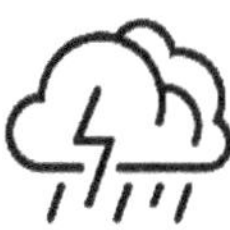

MY 3 MINUTE GRATITUDE JOURNAL

01 **Today I feel**
Tick the face below...

DATE _____ / ___ / ___

TIME _______ : ___

02 **Gratitude.**
I am grateful for...

____

____

____

03 **Complete this sentence**
Today I am looking forward to.......

____

____

____

____

04 **Today is:**

01 Today I feel
Tick the face below...

DATE ___/___/___

TIME _______ : _______

 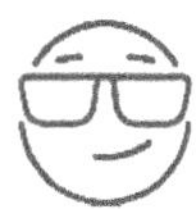    

02 Gratitude.
I am grateful for...

____

____

____

03 Complete this sentence
Today I am looking forward to.......

____

____

____

04 Today is:

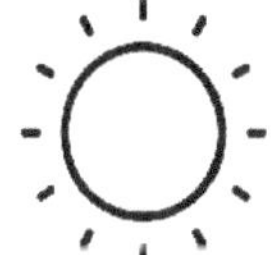  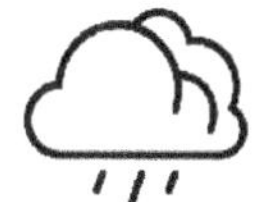 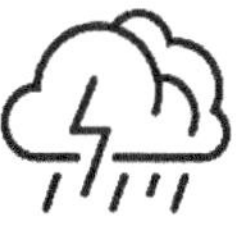  

MY 3 MINUTE
GRATITUDE JOURNAL

Congratulations! You have completed DAY 90. That is an amazing achievement!

01 Moments

What were your favorite 3 things you did over the past 90 days?

1.

2.

3.

02 Be Creative!

Draw a picture or stick a photo here that was a special moment for you over the past 90 days.

90 Day Journal Notes

Write here whatever you feel like. Is there something special you would like to include to complete your journal?

90 Day Journal Notes

____

____

____

____

____

____

____

____

Do you have a photo or picture you would like to include here?

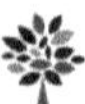

"Nothing new can come into your life unless you are grateful for what you already have"

- Michael Bernard

About the Author

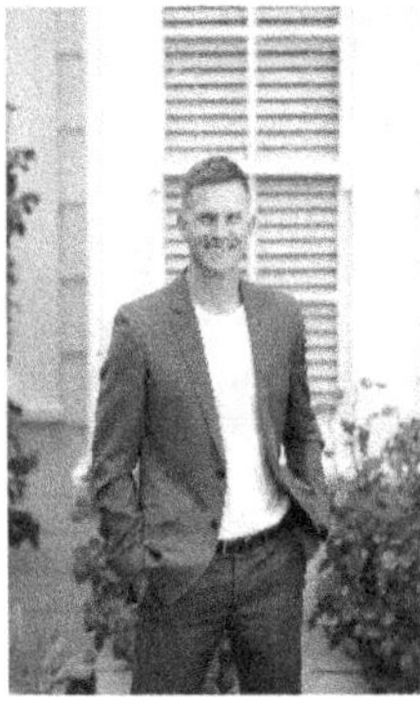

Romney Nelson is a #1 Amazon Best Selling Author and Leading Australian Goal Setting and Habit Development Expert. He commenced his career as a secondary school teacher working in some of the most well-known schools in Australia, including Head of Faculty positions in Oxford and Wimbledon, United Kingdom.

Romney authored his first resource, PE on the GO; a physical education resource for teachers in 2009 and in 2019, he created The Daily Goal Tracker, a powerful and practical resource developed to Create, Track and Achieve your goals. In 2020, Romney became an Amazon Best Selling Author with the release of The Habit Switch. His other books include Magnetic Goals, The Daily Goal Tracker, The 5 Minute Morning Journal and various children's books.